Anti-Inflammatory Essential Oils

18 Best Essential Oil Remedies To Suppress Inflammation and Pain

Tonny M Ford, RN, BSN, PHN.

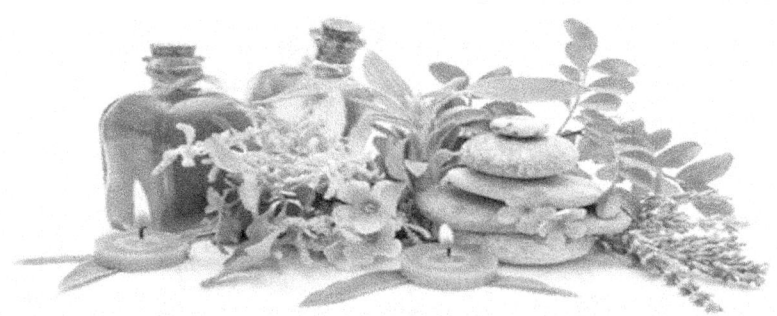

ANTI INFLAMMATORY
Essential
Oils

18 BEST ESSENTIAL OIL REMEDIES TO SUPPRESS INFLAMMATION AND PAIN

TONNY M FORD, RN, BSN, PHN

essentialoilRN.net

for any reparation, damages, or monetary loss due to the information herein, either directly or indirectly.

Respective authors own all copyrights not held by the publisher.

The information herein is offered for informational purposes solely, and is universal as so. The presentation of the information is without contract or any type of guarantee assurance.

The trademarks that are used are without any consent, and the publication of the trademark is without permission or backing by the trademark owner. All trademarks and brands within this book are for clarifying purposes only and are the owned by the owners themselves, not affiliated with this document.

Disclaimer

This book is not intended as a substitute for the medical advice of physicians. The reader should regularly consult a physician in matters relating to his/her health and particularly with respect to any symptoms that may require diagnosis or medical attention.

The information provided in this book is designed to provide helpful information on the subjects discussed. This book is not meant to be used, nor should it be used, to diagnose or treat any medical condition. For diagnosis or treatment of any medical problem, consult your own physician. The publisher and author are not responsible for any specific health or medical needs that may require medical supervision and are not liable for any damages or negative consequences from any treatment, action, application or preparation, to any person reading or following the information in this book. References are provided for informational purposes only and do not constitute endorsement of any websites or other sources. Readers should be aware that the websites listed in this book may change.

This document is geared towards providing exact and reliable information in regards to the topic and issue covered. The publication is sold with the idea that the publisher is not required to render accounting, officially permitted, or otherwise, qualified services. If advice is necessary, legal or professional, a practiced individual in the profession should be ordered.

- From a Declaration of Principles which was accepted and approved equally by a Committee of the American Bar Association and a Committee of Publishers and Associations.

this document is not allowed unless with written permission from the publisher. All rights reserved.

The information provided herein is stated to be truthful and consistent, in that any liability, in terms of inattention or otherwise, by any usage or abuse of any policies, processes, or directions contained within is the solitary and utter responsibility of the recipient reader. Under no circumstances will any legal responsibility or blame be held against the publisher for any reparation, damages, or monetary loss due to the information herein, either directly or indirectly.

Respective authors own all copyrights not held by the publisher.

The information herein is offered for informational purposes solely, and is universal as so. The presentation of the information is without contract or any type of guarantee assurance.

The trademarks that are used are without any consent, and the publication of the trademark is without permission or backing by the trademark owner. All trademarks and brands within this book are for clarifying purposes only and are the owned by the owners themselves, not affiliated with this document.

We highly recommend that you consult a doctor and other trained clinicians before using essentials oils or anything that can affect your health. Your doctor is the only one who knows the true story of your health and can give your better professional help.

Bonus Gift!!

As a way of saying thank you for purchasing our book, we have included a free 140 page exclusive pdf report on **essential oils guide**. We believe that that the value in this report will enrich your life abundantly. As a subscriber, you will the first to get a new free ebooks before anyone else! If you have any questions, please contact us at support@essentialoilrn.net

Click here to download your free bonus ebook

http://www.essentialoilrn.net

Table of Contents

Introduction

Thank you and congratulations for owning the book *"Anti-Inflammatory Essential Oils (18 best essential oil remedies to suppress inflammation and pains.)"*

The number of people living with serious, chronic pain is on the rise. In the USA alone, this condition affects 116 million people every year. Many of whom suffer from debilitating physical pain for up to 60 days or more. This can permanently affect a person's mental and emotional health, and severely affects his/her career, interpersonal relationship with others, and long-term happiness.

Many people are turning to drugs for relief. But dependency on drugs creates more problems than solutions. There's addiction, drug abuse, drug tolerance, rising costs of medications, and suffering through withdrawal symptoms. Furthermore, abusing and misusing medications can become the cause of more chronic pain. This happens when long-term drug use results in blood poisoning, liver and kidney damage, and even multiple organ failure.

Other chronic pain sufferers are turning to drastic measures like surgery. Unless health care providers pinpoint exactly where the source comes from, any kind of operation dealing with chronic pain poses higher-than-normal risks of permanent incapacitation, which can lead to: bone loss, degeneration of soft tissues and the immune system, muscle atrophy, and the onset of all kinds of infections. These surgeries are always expensive, not 100% effective, and may prove fatal for some.

This is the reason why more people are turning to organic and natural measures for chronic pain relief, like using essential oils for their day-to-day therapy.

With the proper instructions, essential oils are safe and non-invasive. Because these are not based on drugs or medications, these are non-addictive, and have very little chances of increasing your tolerance level with every use.

Essential oils are more economical especially if you compare the cost of their daily use versus the cost of regularly using drugs, or undergoing one or more forms of surgery. These are less painful, but equally as effective as other traditional healing methods like: acupuncture, chiropractic, naturopathy, and osteopathy.

Best of all, you can use essential oils on your own, and in the comfort of your home, or anywhere else you desire.

This book contains information as to how you can use essential oils to gain long-term and pain-free existence. Included is a list of pure oils and oil compounds that you can use for specific forms of chronic pain treatment.

This also contains facts about different massages you can try, different forms of aromatherapy, and how to make your own essential oil compounds at home.

Just remember: the information within this book will not cure the cause of your chronic pain. Rather, it will teach you ways on how to ease some or all of its symptoms.

Thank you again for getting the book. I hope this book gives you the relief you need. Enjoy!

Chapter 1: A Few Things to Consider Before Starting

Choosing organic measures as a form of treatment for chronic pain is always a great thing. This means that you are ready to abandon drug-based treatments, and reap the benefits of a safer, healthier, and potentially pain-free lifestyle. Before you embark on this journey though, here are a few things you should do or consider.

1. Always ask your health care provider for the "go" signal, before embarking on any therapy. This is especially true if you are/have:

   - Currently taking powerful drugs for existing medical conditions, or

   - Currently undergoing other forms of therapy, (e.g. chemotherapy, etc.,) or

   - Recently undergone any form of operation, even minor ones (e.g. tooth extraction, etc.)

   - Lactating, pregnant, or trying to conceive

   - Any allergic reaction to oils or oil-based products

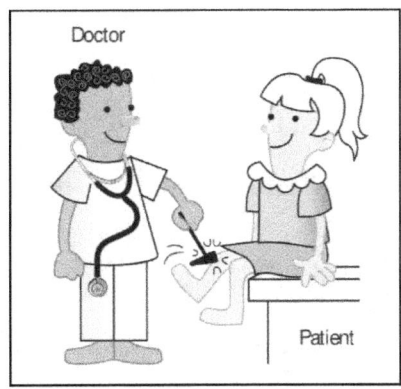

2. If you are practicing self-massage, always do so with recently cleaned and dried skin. This means washing or gently scrubbing clean the intended area with soap and water. Also, having a clean pair of hands to work with limits infection and prevents epidermal damage.

If you are practicing aromatherapy, always make sure your tools are equally clean. Meticulously wash your diffuser *before* and *after* using. You have to remember that mould and mildew can sprout up anywhere, including the nooks and crannies of your machine. Unfortunately, their spores can also become airborne, and bound for your lungs if you are not careful.

3. Take careful note of which oils are safe for massage therapy, and which ones should only be used for aromatherapy. Though both are technically safe to use, massage oils are

developed specifically to be topical or readily absorbable by the skin.

On the other hand, aromatherapy oils should always be diluted prior to use, and only be diffused in the air. These should not be applied directly onto the skin.

4. Use massage-safe oils that work well with your skin. If you can, do a simple skin or patch test. Spray or apply a small amount of oil on your wrist, and rub it gently in. Tie or cover the area with a piece of clean gauze, the let it sit there for 30 to 45 minutes. If you have no allergic reactions to the oil (e.g. you don't experience itchiness, or you don't see rashes forming,) then you can safely use the massage oils.

5. Massages cannot be rushed. A 15-minute massage cannot be compressed into 3 minutes by applying more pressure to the area. This will only lead to more physical damage, and more episodes of chronic pain. So if you are committing to any form of massage, make sure you make enough time for it.

Likewise, the best kind of massage for chronic pain can ultimately lead to restorative sleep. If possible, take a nap after your massage. But a better option is to do your massages right before bedtime so that you can sleep fitfully afterwards.

6. Do not take a warm bath or cold shower immediately after a massage. This can potentially undo all the healthful benefits of your massage, and may even cause muscle tension and cramps. Worse, it may cause the onset of pneumonia especially if your health is already compromised, or you are highly susceptible to colds and flus.

If you must, you should wait for at least an hour before taking a **warm** bath. Better yet, take a quick shower before you get the massage.

7. Avoid any strenuous physical activity immediately after a massage. Wait for an hour or two before doing any heavy lifting or prolonged exercises. This will give your body enough time to regain its equilibrium (e.g. cool down or warm up, depending on the kind of massage,) and prevent possible injuries, especially in the ligaments, muscles, and tendons.

You can exercise first before getting a massage. Then rest for a good 30 minutes afterwards. You can prolong your resting period by taking a quick shower, or a long, hot bath. This will release some tension from your tired muscles.

Practice the various forms of relaxing. Getting a massage is one thing. Being stressed *during* a massage is another. If you are getting a massage, or giving yourself one, it is essential to calm your nerves, and organically ease your stress. You can do this by simply doing a few breathing exercises prior to your massage.

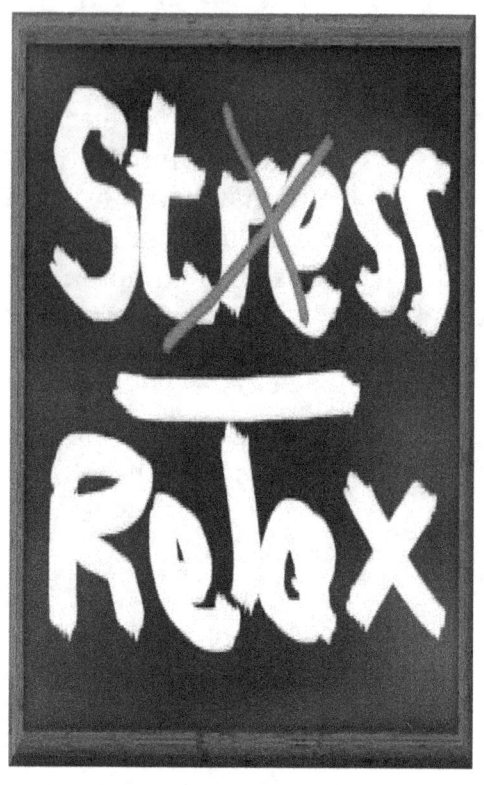

If you feel too tense, it might be a good idea to sleep on it; or at least, take a power nap. A long soak in the bathtub might be a good idea as well, or perform any activity which you find calming, like taking a stroll around the neighbourhood. Forcing the issue will only cause you more harm than good.

For chronic pain treatment, it is best to do the massage after the pain has subsided. Although it sounds counterintuitive, do not massage affected areas during the peak of its pain. You will only damage arteries, nerves, muscles, and veins if you do so. Plus, you will subject yourself to more aches and bruises.

Wait for a couple of minutes after the pain subsides before you massage the area. And always wait until your muscles relax before doing so.

Remember: _therapeutic massage should ease the pain, and not contribute to it_.

8. Create and follow a regular routine for your massages. This will make pain management easier. Try to schedule your daily massages on the same time, with a lot of room afterwards for rest or sleep. Your body will accept the changes you are making faster.

9. Choose a quiet room and a restful space. This is especially beneficial for aromatherapy. According to research, a relaxing ambience can speed up the healing process by almost 100%. It does not have to be an overly silent room, or a large space. Any spot where you can feel completely comfortable will do.

Listening to music or ambient noise (e.g. chirping birds, running water, etc.) is optional. Any kind of relaxing music will do, as long as you keep the volume at a low setting.

Additionally, there are studies that show that a slightly darkened room helps people relax faster. So, if you are at home, partially closing the blinds, or doing your massages at dawn or any time after dusk would be beneficial to your health.

10. The intensity and the duration of the massage should always be of your choosing. This is especially true if someone else is giving you the massage. A good massage should ease your pains. This would also depend on how high or low your threshold of pain is.

For some people, "hard" massages work well in easing muscle tension pain. Others prefer gentler forms of massage techniques. (See Chapter 2 for the different types of massages.)

In any case, you should ask the person giving you the massage to stop once pain sets in. If you are doing this by yourself, always stop when you feel the pain. Let the affected area rest a bit (for around 5 to 30 minutes) before continuing. If the pain persists, stop immediately. Consult your health care provider at the most convenient time.

Chapter 2: What Is Chronic Pain?

Definition

Chronic pain is any kind of physical discomfort that lasts for more than 2 weeks. This is the kind of pain that persists for days, months, years, and even decades after the first incidence. It is very likely that chronic pain does not respond well to any conventional forms of treatment, like: over-the-counter analgesics or pain relievers.

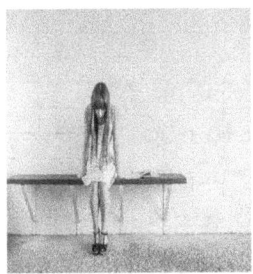
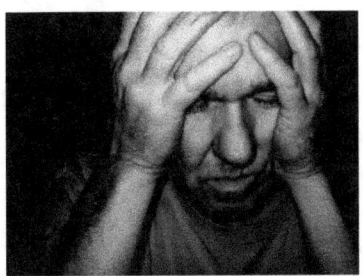
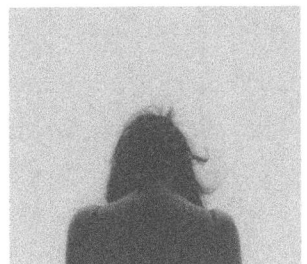

Unlike acute pain which disappears after a while (usually after the initial injury heals,) chronic pain can continue for a long time, even and especially when there are no longer any visible signs of bodily damage. In many cases, it will outlast the course of the initial ailment, disease, or injury by a hundred-fold.

A person suffering from this condition can feel aches, soreness, or agonizing pain returning intermittently, or at regular intervals, or at the most inopportune moments.

Some cases are triggered when:

- A person experiences sudden, regular, or intermittent shifts in temperature, climate, or weather. For example:

  - While the person is outside, weather changes from intense rain to sweltering heat in a matter of minutes. Or,

  - When a person spends all day in an air-conditioned office, then suddenly steps out to a dry, humid, and/or hot day, and vice versa.

There are studies that show that this kind of pain is due to barometric pressure in the body not adjusting quickly enough to temperature change. Blood vessels contract and expand painfully, usually in an unsynchronized pattern.

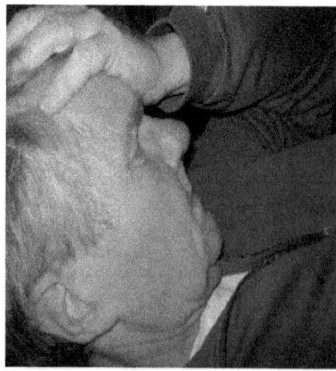 This usually affects smaller blood vessels found in the respiratory system, and those that connect to the brain. People who are highly susceptible to headaches and migraines usually suffer from chronic pain

due to sudden shifts in temperature.

The same holds true for people who have one or more types of respiratory ailments or diseases, like:

- Acute respiratory distress syndrome
- Asthma
- Bacterial pneumonia
- Bronchitis
- Chronic obstructive pulmonary disorder
- Cystic fibrosis
- Emphysema
- Head and neck cancer
- Lower respiratory tract infection
  - Pneumocystis
  - Pneumonia, and all its complications
  - Severe acute respiratory syndrome
  - Tuberculosis
- Lung cancer
  - *Adenocarcinoma* of the lungs
  - Kaposi's sarcoma
  - Large cell lung cancer
  - Lymphoma
  - Melanoma
  - Pleural *mesothelioma*
  - Squamous cell carcinoma of the lung
  - Small cell lung cancer
- Pulmonary arterial hypertension
- Pulmonary embolism
- Pulmonary edema

- Pulmonary haemorrhage
- Upper respiratory tract infection
  - Laryngitis
  - Pharyngitis
  - Sinusitis
  - Tonsillitis

Sudden shifts in temperature also trigger pain in people who have or are susceptible to arthritis, gout, and rheumatism.

- A person shifts to potentially damaging postures or positions. This often leads to chronic back aches, stiffness of the lower lumbar area, and even unnatural curvature of the spine. For example:

  - A person tries to improperly lift heavy objects. Or,

  - A person spends all day hunched over a table while working. Or,

  - A person who overuses or abuses specific muscle groups, like forearms, arms, and shoulders while body building.

This kind of pain usually stems from abnormal wears and tears of the musculature, resulting in microscopic or cell-deep damage. Often referred to as *muscle strain(s)* or *pulled muscle(s),* this condition can afflict any part of the body, but is common in the longer muscles of the hamstring, lower back, neck, and shoulders.

Extreme cases of muscle strain may necessitate corrective surgery to ease chronic pain and return full mobility to the affected area. Early detection of this condition can limit or prevent further episodes of chronic pain.

- A person is constantly exposing himself/herself to harmful stimuli. For example:

    o A person spends inordinate amount of time under the sun with no or little skin protection. Or,

    o A person is constantly exposed to toxic fumes, like exhaust gases from vehicles, chemical vapors, hot steam, and factory gasses (etc.). Or,

    o A person constantly or chronically suffers from (emotional, mental, or physical) stress.

Any kind of stimulus, whether beneficial or harmful, affects the body from the macro down to the micro level. Naturally, harmful stimuli like exposing your skin to too much sun have lasting effects because it takes time for the body to heal from any kind of injury.

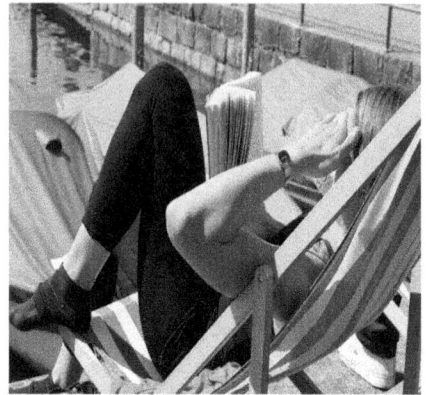

Too much solar or ultraviolet radiation exposure can cause:

- Damage to the eyes or eyesight, which can lead to chronic pain behind the eyes
- Premature aging of the skin, due to loss of epidermal elasticity
- Skin rashes, sunburns, and other blemishes
- Skin cancer and/or chronic pain in the epidermis or dermis

The earliest stages of basal cell skin cancer, squamous cell skin cancer, and Bowen's disease usually start with feeling chronic pain for 2 weeks (or more) just underneath the epidermis (dermis,) particularly on the ears, back, face, hands, scalp, and shoulders.

These are followed by the appearance of lumps or discoloured patches on the skin, which can become sensitive or tender to the touch.

Other harmful stimuli like toxic fumes and stress can also cause microscopic damage to internal organs, particularly the kidneys and liver, in the muscles of the circulatory and respiratory systems, and within the gastrointestinal lining. These conditions lead to the steady deterioration of physical health, which in turn, increase the risk of deep, persistent chronic pain elsewhere in the body.

In this regard, prevention and/or early detection are the best ways to keep the pain at bay.

Various studies also verify that few people experience the same level of pain. It is more likely that the discomfort escalates over time as the afflicted person's health declines.

Chronic pain may range from tolerable soreness, to tenderness of bones, joints and muscles, to debilitating and crippling outbreaks. Many cases do not have single source points, while others may stem from initial injuries, like:

- Allergic reactions
- Broken bones
- Bruises
- Burns and scalds
- Cuts and grazes
- Dislocation of fingers, toes, and other limbs
- Eye injuries
- Insect and/or animal bites
- Infections (any form)
- Lacerations

- Minor head injuries
- Minor injuries to the hands, arms and legs
- Muscle Strains
- Sprains
- Superficial abrasions

Others are triggered or exacerbated by existing medical conditions, such as:

- AIDS or Acquired Immune Deficiency Syndrome
- Cancer, all forms
- Cardiovascular ailments and diseases, all forms
- Congenital diseases that lead to the curvature of the spine, or damage to the spinal cord, such as:
  o Multiple scoliosis
  o Osteoarthritis
- Depression
- Diabetes, especially if the person has a naturally slow healing capacity
- Fatigue or exhaustion, chronic
- Fibromyalgia syndrome
- Gallbladder disease
- Gastro-intestinal disease
  - Acid reflux syndrome
  - Obstruction of the bowels
  - Stomach ulcers
- Lack of sleep and/or sleep disturbances, chronic
- Major physical injuries that fail to heal properly

- o Brain or head injuries
- o Nerve damage
- o Spinal damage, such as: degenerative spinal disc disease
- Permanent nerve damage
- Respiratory ailments and diseases
- Rheumatoid arthritis
- Spinal pain due to years of poor posture
- Tissue damage
- Traumatic injury that leads to psychological and physical distress
- Weight management issues

  - o Being obese or overweight puts constant strain on the spine, the muscles of the back, and the joints of the knees. This is especially dangerous if the person packs on the pounds in a relatively short amount of time. Being obese or overweight usually leads to a number of chronic pain issues, including pain from compromised internal organs.

  - o Being chronically underweight due to any form of eating disorder can permanently damage bones, internal organs, and muscles too. Two of the most common examples are: anorexia nervosa, and bulimia nervosa.

  - o Uncontrollable weight gain or weight loss, usually due to another medical condition, such as the onset of cancer, tuberculosis, gastrointestinal diseases, hyperthyroidism, and liver damage can be root causes of long-term chronic pain.

- Weight gain or weight loss in a relatively short amount of time, usually due to obsessive weight lifting or body sculpting, and excessive crash dieting can damage muscle groups and internal organs in a hurry. Chronic pain is usually an indicator that the body is not adapting well to the sudden changes.

According to research, 38% to 44% of chronic pain sufferers have various medical conditions that snowball into different levels and stages of bodily aches. Suffering from chronic pain alone can trigger:

- Decrease in appetite. According to research, chronic pain sufferers will often turn away from food. Hunger, thirst, and the body's need for nutrition all take the back seat when it comes to dealing with crippling or debilitating pain. In turn, poor nutrition can lead to the weakening of one's immune system, and make a person more susceptible to:

  - Cold sores
  - Common colds or influenza
  - Fatigue
  - Infections, all kinds
  - Recurring episodes of swollen lymph glands and/or nodes

- o Recurring and escalating soreness in the joints and muscles

- Emotional and mental stress. This can lead to depression and other graver forms of mental disorders. This can also be the root cause of chronic migraines.

- Irreversible damage to internal organs and the surrounding tissues. It is quite normal for a person to find ways to ease chronic pain. This may include regularly popping pain killers, or numbing the pain by consuming alcohol.

  Unfortunately, overmedicating on pain killers and overconsumption of alcohol can damage liver and kidneys, and/or burn holes (ulcers) in the stomach or intestinal lining. All of which can lead to more damaging and painful medical conditions.

- Muscles atrophy, especially in the limbs, neck, and shoulders. When a person wilfully limits the use of afflicted body parts due to pain, the muscles within shrink or shrivel up due to lack of use. This puts more strain on ligaments and tendons which hold muscles and bones together. Any minute tear in the muscles, ligaments, and tendons due to muscular atrophy can trigger chronic, deep-seated pain. This can also lead to a steadily decline in physical flexibility and mobility. Overall stamina and strength is likewise compromised.

Diagnosis

Pain is quite subjective. There is no accurate way of gauging pain level, or where exactly it originates. Two people may experience the same intensity of pain in the same possible location, but their descriptions of it may be worlds apart. Even the most advanced diagnostic machines can offer little help or support if the person suffering from chronic pain cannot articulate exactly how excruciating it is, or where its possible source may be.

Also, the source of chronic pain may become indeterminate, even if there seems to be a possible origin of the discomfort. For example: a person underwent corrective knee surgery decades ago.

- He may still feel chronic pain in that particular area due to tendons and muscles not healing correctly. Or,
- The pain may stem from an undetected or untreated infection of the ligaments of the knee cap after the operation. Or,
- The corrective surgery caused bone loss in the joints of the thigh and shin bones, where the knee is connected. Or,
- It could stem from a different and unrelated disease altogether.

According to research, the reported range of discomfort includes:

- Bone deep ache
- Burning sensation
- Chopping or slicing sensation
- Cramps, or any similar sensation
- Deep persistent ache in the internal organs
- Dull ache, or hollow but painful feeling
- Grating or grinding sensation (especially in the bones and joints)
- Malfunctioning or non-functioning of limbs or specific body parts
- Numbness followed by immobility, or muscles feeling heavy or leaden
- Radiating pain, or pain that seems to spread outwards
- Severe pain that cause partial or full bodily paralysis
- Sharp prickling sensation
- Stabbing sensation
- Stiffening of the muscles, or stiffness of particular body parts
- Tender or sore to the touch
- Tingling sensation, followed by numbness or pain
- Tightness, particularly in the torso area
- Throbbing sensation and/or pulsating pain
- Uncontrollable tics or twitches, usually in the face

Proper chronic pain diagnosis is further compounded by the fact that people have their own unique genetic makeup. Some people may respond well to certain treatments, while others show no improvement at all. Worse, some people's health may be compromised when subjected to the same treatments.

Another obstacle to correctly diagnosing chronic pain is people's propensity to ignore or tolerate it for the longest time possible. Some people just want to avoid going to the doctor's office (due to lack of finances or insurance coverage,) while others force themselves to believe that the discomfort will go away on its own. Of course, there are those who self-medicate, relying mostly on over-the-counter pain relievers or powerful (and sometimes illegal) drugs.

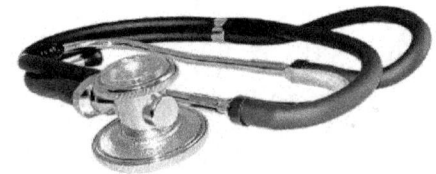

More Common Forms of Chronic Pain Treatment

The foremost goal for chronic pain treatment is to find the cause, heal it, and improve the state of the afflicted body parts. 89% of the time though, health care providers cannot find the actual source of discomfort, especially when the visible wounds or obvious illness has already healed.

Chronic pain is an indicator that something else is off, and it may or may not be related to the initial medical condition or injury.

It should also be noted that an average person may suffer from one or more forms of bodily injury (both minor and major) at the same time, or one after the other.

If the primary goal is not met, the secondary goal is to simply lessen the intensity or frequency of the discomfort, so that the person can have a better (or improved) quality of life.

Aside from taking medications and drugs, some of the most common chronic pain treatments are:

- Acupuncture, an ancient form of treatment that involves inserting fine needles into the meridian or chi points of the body. This helps manipulate the flow of good energy into the body, while releasing the trapped energy that may be causing the person discomfort or sickness. Acupuncture is still very much practiced today.

- Application of hot and/or cold compress

  - Heat opens up the blood vessels which promote better blood flow to ligaments, muscles, and tendons. Applying hot compress to body parts improves the flexibility of tendons, relaxes the muscles, and lessens the strain on tendons.

  - Cold slows down the flow of blood to any recent injury/injuries. Applying cold compress on specific body parts can reduce swelling, limit inflammation, and numb down the pain.

- Low impact, cardiovascular exercises. Exercises like these do not cure chronic pain, but can help improve flexibility of the spine, and muscular/joint mobility. These are essential when promoting better blood flow or lymphatic movement throughout the body. Like:

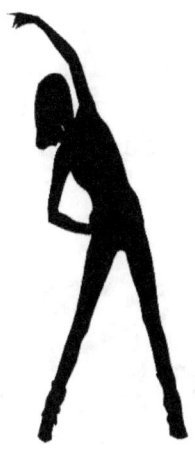

- o Ballroom dancing
  - o Golf
  - o Hiking or exploring
  - o Low-impact water aerobics / water dancing
  - o Pilates for beginners
- o Stationary cycling or rowing
- o Step aerobics
- o *Tai chi*
- o Walking or brisk walking
- o Using the elliptical machine or the Stairmaster
- o Yoga for beginners

- Medications, may involve consuming various forms of drugs, food supplements, and any type of liquid-based medication. For example:

- Drug pumps or infusion pumps. Pain medication is directly administered to the *intrathecal space* or the fluid that surrounds the spinal cord. This is recommended only to people who do not respond well to most oral medications. This is considered as an invasive form of treatment, which necessitates surgery to implant the "system" which includes a pump and a catheter.

o Mild pain relievers or analgesic (oral medications.) These are common, over-the-counter drugs that are readily available anywhere. Some of these include:

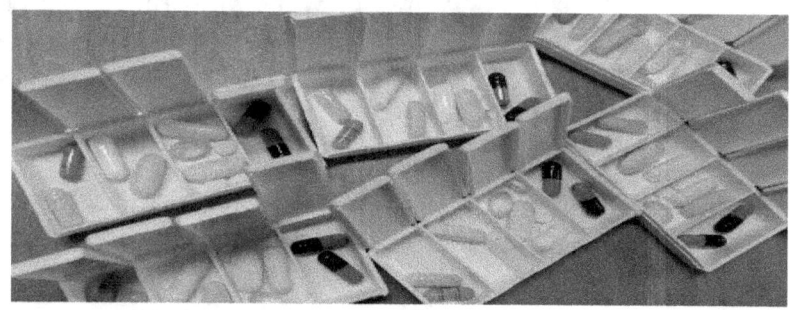

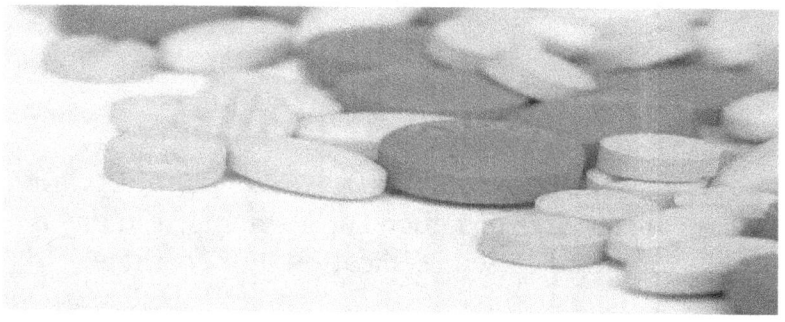

o COX-2 inhibitors (*celecoxib, etoricoxib,* and *rofecoxib,* etc.)
- Non-steroid based anti-inflammatory drugs (e.g. *salicylates,* etc.)
- *Opioid* (e.g. *codeine, dihydromorphione, hydrocodone, morphine, oxycodone, pethidine,* etc.)
- Paracetamol / *acetaminophen* (e.g. aspirin, etc.)
- Specific agents for chronic neuropathic pain (e.g. antidepressants, anticonvulsants, etc.)

- Topical or systemic analgesia (creams, gels, ointments, etc.)

- Nerve blockers. Patients are regularly given local anaesthetics, or steroid-based injections to provide relief, albeit temporarily.)

o Psychotherapy is a form of treatment that uses mental exercises, instead of medical or surgical means. This is a highly subjective, because episodes of chronic pain are influenced by how the brain processes pain signals, and the person's inherent coping strategies. The most common psychotherapies for persistent pain are:

- Relaxation techniques. This involves concentrating while doing breathing exercises. This helps relax muscles, and ease pain.

Relaxation also helps the person rest or sleep easier, which makes the body heal faster.

- Age progression or regression. This is a device wherein the person is encouraged to think ahead or think back in time when the pain did not exist. Then the person "instructs" his/her future or past self how to deal with the condition.

- Altered focus. This entails focusing on any non-painful part of the body to alter the sensations in the afflicted area.

- Counting. Silently counting helps distract the mind from the messages sent by the pain receptors. Patients are instructed to count breaths, cracks in the pavement, passing cars, etc.

    - Deep muscle relaxation. This involves tensing and relaxing the muscles in 10 to 15 second successions, making it easy to feel the difference between the relaxed state and the painful state.

    - Dissociation. This relies on the person's ability to separate normally connected thoughts in order to distance oneself from the pain.

- Distraction. The person attempts to move attention away from the pain.

- Hypnosis. This is rather extreme, but some people who have undergone this process say that their perception of pain have lessened to some degree. Hypnosis can be done with the help of a trained hypnosis, or by oneself.

- Mental analgesia and mental anaesthesia. This entails imagining applying or injecting powerful drugs, anaesthetics, or cooling packs on or into the afflicted area.

- Positive imagery. Focusing your energy into something pleasant or happy.

- Sensory splitting. This entails dividing the painful sensations into different components, and focusing on each separately. For example: if you are experiencing pain in your lower lumbar area that feels hot or warm to the touch, you focus healing thoughts on the heat first, then on the pain when the heat "subsides."

- Symbolic imagery. This entails creating symbols to represent the pain. For example: a loud blaring noise symbolizes the pain. The person symbolically turns the noise down, so that the pain lessens as well.

- Transfer, also called pain movement. This involves altering the pain sensations by trying to transfer the some into the non-afflicted areas. Apparently, the shared sensation is easier to bear.

- Visual imagery. The person chooses pictures, sounds, thoughts, or videos that provide pleasant and relaxing experiences, in an attempt to mask or lessen pain.

- Surgery.

  - Corrective surgery. This is usually done when health care providers actually trace the source of the patient's discomfort. This could range anywhere from readjusting bone structure, to surgically stapling torn muscles, and more. However, this only yields 30% to 50% success rate. Sometimes, surgery causes more or different forms of chronic pain.

o Electrical stimulation, also known as neuro-stimulators. Using a machine or device, this form of therapy sends out mild electrical impulses into the spine that will hinder or slow down the pain messages the body sends to the brain. This produces a numbing effect. Though not technically as invasive as the other forms of surgery, this kind of treatment still needs to be done under the supervision of a health care professional or a trained professional.

o Radiofrequency *neuro ablation*. This is a relatively expensive operation using heat from radiofrequency electrodes, wherein the surgeon literally burns away some of the nerve endings of pain receptors. This limits the pain signals that go to the brain. It can only be applied on the back, coccyx (tailbone,) neck, and sacrum area (the triangular bone found at the base of the spine.)

The level/intensity of relief depends greatly on the patient's overall health. Also, the length of relief is only for a year or less.

- Massage therapy and/or physical therapy. Massage therapy is the manual manipulation of the soft tissues of the body, particularly the connective tissues, joints, ligaments, muscles, and tendons. This is a form of non-invasive treatment which attempts to build or recondition the muscles and nerves by promoting better blood flow to the affected areas.

  This is usually done by putting mild or sustained pressure on key points all over the body. Fingers and hands are the primary tools for massages, though you can also use elbows, forearms, knees and feet.

  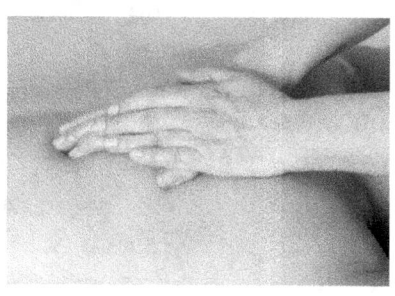

  - Aromatherapy is a form of relaxing massage that utilizes aromatic plant oils and other compounds as a way of improving the person's mental and physical condition by:

    - Fighting a broad spectrum of bacterial, fungal, and viral infections on the skin, hair and nails

    - Improving the person's mood

- Promoting faster healing of wounds

- Promoting restive sleep

- Reducing inflammation

- Rejuvenating skin

- Soothing superficial skin irritations

- Stimulating better blood circulation, especially to the limbs

o Acupressure (a combination of acupuncture and pressure) is a form of massage that puts pressure on the acupuncture points of body. Needles are not used, but fingers, hands and elbows are.

o *Anma* massage originated from Japan. This is a more vigorous form of physical therapy that involves: kneading the muscles hard, rubbing, shaking, and tapping joints and bones. This is usually done through clothing, hence the need for energetic manipulation.

o *Ashiatsu*

Practitioners use their feet to massage parts of the body. The arches, heel, and surface of the feet, combined with the weight of the practitioner place enough pressure on the large muscles of the body. This kind of massage is best done on the back area (not on the spine,) and the back of the calves. It is not ideal for other parts of the body.

Balinese massage is a more relaxing form of massage. It involves gentle muscle kneading, skin folding, stroking, and rolling motions near or around joints. Using hot or heated volcanic stones is optional.

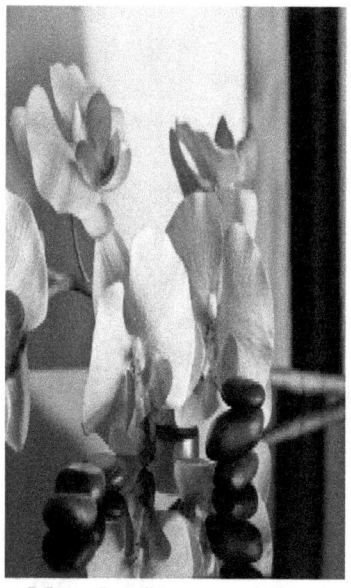

- o Bowen technique involves making short, rolling strokes on the large muscles to promote better blood flow. This is usually done to relive muscle tension and strains (e.g. leg cramps.)

- o *Breema* massage is a self-massage technique which involves more stretching than actual tissue manipulation. This can be done almost anywhere, just as long as there is enough space to move about.

o *Champissage* massage is a series of gently exercises, usually focusing on muscles from the neck up. It involves making rolling or kneading movements using the fingers on chakra points on the brow, crown, nape, neck, and throat.

o Craniosacral therapy is another gentle kind of massage that involves releasing tension on the face, parts of the skull, pelvis, and spine.

o Foot massage involves various forms of massages, all of which are directed to the soles of the feet, toes, ankles, and sometimes on calves. (This would depend on the extent of the services being offered

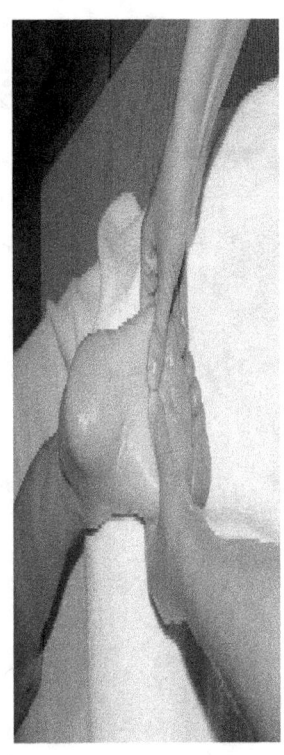

by the practitioner.)

- Immersion. This is a massage technique that requires immersing the whole body, or parts of the body in relaxing liquids or semi-liquids. This can be as simple as soaking in a tub of warm, soapy water with bath salts, or in mineral-rich mud baths.

  - *Balneo* therapy refers to the therapeutic bathing in thermal springs that havr naturally occurring oils and minerals.

- Mud bath therapy refers to the soaking or being covered with mineral-rich, naturally occurring moist earth. These are prevalent in lava-prone territory where the mud contains inordinate amounts of salt and other minerals.

  - *Thalasso* therapy refers to the therapeutic bathing in ocean or marine water. These too contain naturally occurring oils and salt.

  - Water immersion (not to be confused with Water Cure or Hydrotherapy.) A person soaks specific body parts into aromatic water. This helps soften the skin and allows faster absorption of minerals into the pores of the skin.

o Manual lymphatic drainage's main goal is to reduce swelling of the lymph nodes. Aside from placing gentle rolling motions on the affected area, the practitioner also makes long strokes following the path of veins and nerves. This is supposed help improve a person's immune functions while promoting better elimination of waste products.

o Reflexology works on the principle of massaging the organic reflexes found in the hands and feet, in relevance to the other organs of the body. For example: pressing qi (chi) points at the base of the thumb can ease chronic lower back problems. Reflexology can also be administered on to oneself.

o Swedish massage is a lengthy kind of massage. It undergoes 5 traditional stages or "strokes." These are: *effleurage* (sliding stroke,) *petrissage* (kneading movement,) *tapotement* (tapping motions,) *friktion* (friction or vigorous rubbing,) and *vibrationer* (vibration, often using a machine.) Swedish massage promotes restive sleep afterwards.

- Thai massage (Nuad Boran or Nuat Thai) is a deep full body massage which usually starts from the feet up. Long strokes are supposed to unblock the energy or chi lines of the body.

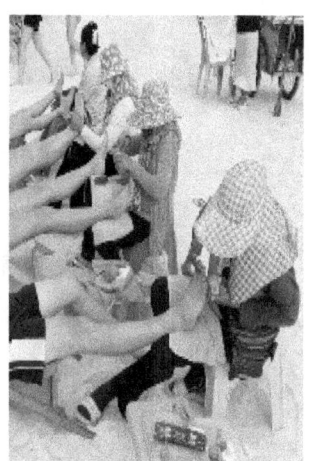

Benefits of Massage Therapy for Chronic Pain Treatment

1. Manual manipulation of muscles, especially soft rolling motions followed by long, gentle strokes, helps the body release serotonin, which is a naturally occurring chemical compound. It plays a major part in promoting happiness and improving one's mood. It also helps lessen feelings of anxiety.

2. A good massage promotes deep, restorative sleep. This lessens the frequency and intensity of chronic pain. Plus, sleep promotes healing in the cellular level.

3. People who chronically suffer from arthritis, fibromyalgia, osteoporosis, and rheumatism show significant improvement in mobility when they receive regular massages. They also claim to gain better strength and flexibility in the affected areas. Some report a noticeable decrease in pain level and frequency.

4. Getting regular massages help reduce and/or prevent chronic muscular tension. This happens when the muscles of the body contract but would not release quickly or at all. Unlike cramps which give out intense pain signals to the brain, muscular tension is quite low-key.

   At the most, the person feels heaviness or stiffness in and around the affected area. Sometimes, the person would feel tightness in the muscles, or what many people refer to as "knots." This commonly happens to overworked muscles from the shoulders up. Sometimes, knots can form in the jaw and nape area too.

When untreated, muscular tension can cause stiffness in the surrounding muscles, slight immobility, and tension headaches.

5. Getting regular massages improves lymphatic drainage. When lymph nodes or glands are surgically removed (e.g. for mastectomy or other cancer-related operations,) it causes waste products from the cardiovascular system (fat cells or plaques in the blood) to build up in veins and arteries.

   Too much plaque can clog smaller veins and arteries until blockages form. This causes blood poisoning and poor blood circulation, which can lead to heart attacks and strokes.

6. Massage therapy can be used as a preventive measure, especially before and after sports training or serious physical workout. Massages help loosen muscles, while strengthening tendons and ligaments by keeping these flexible and pliable. Massages can also help warm up and/or cool down muscles.

7. Massage therapy is an essential component in any stress management program. It does not matter if it's emotional, mental or physical. Gently massaging specific muscles groups can ease tension brought about by stress. Aromatherapy and other forms of massage therapy (e.g. immersion, see page 20) work well as natural and organic stress relievers.

8. Regular massage therapy proves to be quite beneficial to people who suffer from:

   - Alzheimer's disease, some symptoms only
   - Anxiety attacks
   - Asthma
   - Bursitis
   - Back, leg and neck pain
   - Cancer, some symptoms only
   - Carpal tunnel syndrome or repetitive strain on arm ligaments and tendons
   - Chronic fatigue syndrome
   - Depression
   - Dislocations
   - Fibromyalgia
   - Gastrointestinal disorders, some symptoms only
   - Kyphosis
   - Headaches
   - Insomnia
   - Multiple sclerosis
   - Muscle strains
   - Muscle tension and spasm

- Palliative care
- Parkinson's disease, some symptoms only
- Post-surgical rehabilitation
- Scoliosis
- Sports injuries
- Sprains
- Stress and stress-related symptoms
- Tendinitis
- Whiplash

9. Massage therapy is non-invasive, non-addictive, and very affordable. It can be administered to almost anyone, from any age group. It can also be given to people who suffer from any kind of chronic pain, on almost all parts of the body.

Chapter 3: What Are Essential Oils?

Essential oils for chronic pain treatment are usually made from plant oils, or from the "essence" of their main ingredient(s.) For example: rose essential oil is derived directly from distilled, crushed rose petals, while peanut oil is derived from cooking, then processing peanuts.

There are many kinds of essential oil base.

- Absolutes. Also sometimes called pure, this is the most fragrant of all oil bases, simply because these are extracted from one main ingredient only. Absolutes also contain the highest amounts of plant fiber, colorants, and organic waxes.

  Part of the purification processing of absolute oil bases is solvent (hexane) extraction. This means that trace elements of solvent may be found in the oils. This makes it less-than-ideal to use as topical solutions or in air diffusers.

  However, absolute essential oil bases are regularly used in tiny quantities to perfume candles and potpourri. These should never be incorporated in food items and drinks.

- CO_2, or carbon dioxide extracts. Similar to absolutes, CO_2 essential oil bases undergo the same processing sans the solvent. This makes these oil bases ideal for topical applications (e.g. in creams, lotions, and soaps, etc.) and aromatherapy.

These should never be incorporated in food items and drinks.

- Organic extracts. Instead of hexane, this type of base oil is purified using naturally occurring alcohol and fixed oils. This is one of the safer options for topical applications and aromatherapy.

  These can be incorporated in food items and drinks, but only in moderate amounts. Most organic extracts use common pantry ingredients like: almond oil, avocado oil, grapeseed oil, groundnut oil, and even olive oil.

- Hydrosols. These are actually the liquid (or water) by-product of the essential oil distillation process. Many hydrosols only contain less than 10% of its source essential oil. These work well in most diffusers.

  These should never be incorporated in food items and drinks.

Therapeutic Essential Oils and Their Uses

You can use essential oils by themselves or you can combine these with other essential oils. You can mix and match your blends, depending on what kind of chronic pain you want to treat, or what kind of restful fragrance you want to play with. Here is a breakdown of some of the essential oils in the market.

Chamomile. German chamomile.

Pros: chamomile extracts contain compounds that have anti-inflammatory properties.

Best for: easing muscle cramps, spasms, and abnormal or irregular muscle contractions. These are also great for easing headaches and migraines, as well as pain brought about by PMS or pre-menstrual syndrome.

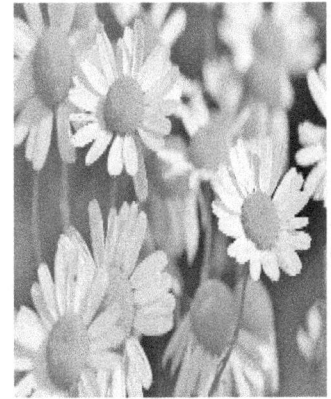

Massage oils with chamomile are considered "mild." These can be used on almost all parts of the body, including the head and the face.

Cons: massage oils with chamomile extracts are not recommended for people with ragweed allergies or flower/seed sensitivities. These are not recommended for very young children, pregnant women, and lactating mothers.

Clove. Clove buds only. Do not use essential oils that contain clove bark, leaves, or roots. These are skin irritants, and may cause painful rashes. Check product labels.
Pros: has anti-inflammatory and anesthetic properties. It can help improve circulation and stimulate metabolism.

Best for: treating chronic pain in the circulatory, cardiovascular, and gastrointestinal systems, especially in the chest area, the back, and the midsection.

Cons: clove essential oil is potent. Use only upon the advice of your health care provider.

Eucalyptus.

Pros: eucalyptus leaves have analgesic and anti-inflammatory properties. Massage oils made from eucalyptus also have organic liniment-like qualities.

Best for: easing chronic muscle pain, fatigue, and muscle tension in the back area, shoulders, and the limbs. These also help ease nerve and chronic deep tissue pain in the chest area (pectorals) and the midsection (abdominal muscles.) Eucalyptus oils are often used as pre-workout rubs.

Cons: because of its strong liniment-like scent and properties, these oils are not recommended to people who have fragrance allergies or sensitivities. These should also be used in small doses. Also, eucalyptus massage oils are not recommended for facial use, particularly near or around the eyes and nose.

Fennel. Fennel bulb, fronds and seeds.

Pros: has mild anti-inflammatory and anti-spasmodic properties.

Best for: mild cases of chronic pain. This help relax muscles and nerves, particularly in the gastrointestinal and reproductive areas.

Cons: Though considered safe, health care providers still do not recommend fennel oil to very young children, pregnant women and lactating mothers.

Frankincense.

Pros: frankincense essential oils have anti-inflammatory and sedative properties. This helps alleviate physical stress, and relieve muscle pains. Frankincense can also spur cell rejuvenation. It helps promote hair root growth, and keep nails looking shiny.

Best for: facial and full body massages. This reduces fine lines, scars, and wrinkles. It is a valuable aid to reducing or lightening
the appearance of stretch marks. This can also be used to ease some of the symptoms of arthritis and rheumatism.
It can promote better circulatory and gastro-intestinal functions. Because of its fragrant nature, this is often used to cure insomnia or promote better sleep.

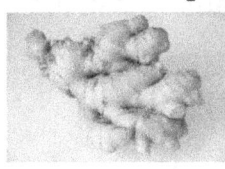 **Cons:** frankincense essential oils are highly fragrant. These are not recommended to people who have fragrance allergies or sensitivities. These should not be administered to very young children, pregnant women, and lactating mothers.

Ginger.

Pros: has anti-rheumatic, antiseptic, anti-spasmodic, and astringent properties.

Best for: easing arthritic and rheumatic pain, especially on the back, the limbs, and phalanges (fingers and toes.) Ginger-based essential oils can also relieve pain by organically providing heat. This works particularly well with sprains, pulled tendons, and damaged ligaments.

Cons: health care providers do not recommend administering ginger-based essential oils to very young children, pregnant women, and lactating mothers. Also, this is not suitable for people who are heat-sensitive, or have existing skin conditions like: sunburns, scratches, open wounds, etc.

Helichrysum **flower.**

Pros: contains analgesic, anti-coagulant, anti-inflammatory, anti-microbial, antiseptic, and antispasmodic properties. Reports say that the relief this provides is almost instantaneous.

Best for: severe arthritic and rheumatic pain. This is also ideal for long-term chronic pain in the lower lumbar area, and the joints of the body.

This helps detoxify the body, as this neutralizes the effects of alcohol, caffeine, and nicotine.

Cons: because of its anti-coagulant properties, this is not recommended to people who had just undergone any form of surgery.

Helichrysum essential oil is also one of the most expensive oils in the market. It is not readily available in most stores.

This is not recommended to very young children, pregnant women, and lactating mothers. This is also not recommended to people with flower extract and/or fragrance allergies and sensitivities.

Juniper. Juniper berries.

Pros: has antispasmodic properties which makes these ideal for backaches, bone aches, leg cramps, joint pains, muscle tension, nerve pains, and basically all forms of muscular cramps. It also has anti-rheumatic properties.

Best for: easing some of the symptoms of muscle strains, and provide relief from arthritis, gout, and rheumatism. Juniper essential oils can ease stomach cramps, PMS, and even chronic tightening of the chest.

When used correctly, it can help relieve swelling of the joints and lymph glands/nodes.

Cons: this must only be used in small amounts, and never on young children, pregnant women, and lactating mothers.

Lavender.

Pros: lavender flower extracts contain anti-inflammatory, anti-microbial, and sedative properties.

Best for: a wide range of ailments – from headaches, to cramps, to muscle tension, and even arthritic pain. It is relatively safe to administer on children 5 years old and above, the infirm, and the elderly.

Lavender oil is considered as one of the lightest and mildest massage oils. It does not heat up when applied on the skin, and it easily permeates through the epidermis without leaving that oily feeling afterwards.

Cons: because of its distinctive scent, lavender oil is not recommended to people who have fragrance allergies or sensitivities.

Marjoram. Sweet marjoram. Wild marjoram.

Pros: This herb naturally contains strong analgesic, antibacterial, antiseptic, and antispasmodic properties.

Best for: this works well with almost all kinds of chronic gastrointestinal chronic pain. This makes it perfect for stomach aches, stomach cramps, and even PMS.

Marjoram essential oils ease symptoms of chronic migraines. These help ease deep pain in the bones like: arthritis and osteoporosis. In small doses, it can also headaches, colds, coughs, insomnia, muscle fatigue, and stress.

Cons: Though considered safe, health care providers do not recommend administering marjoram oils to very young children, pregnant women, and lactating mothers.

People with basil allergies or herb sensitivities should also steer clear of this essential oil.

Peppermint. Spearmint. Water mint.

Pros: Organic peppermint contains menthol, *menthone* and *menthyl esters*. These have analgesic, anti-inflammatory, and antiseptic properties.

Best for: joint, muscle, and nerve pains. This is commonly used in foot spas and leg massages. Peppermint essential oils also have liniment properties which can ease headaches and migraines. This has also been traditionally used to treat bowel spasms, headaches, nausea, PMS, and mild stomach aches.

Cons: because of its strong liniment qualities, this should not be administered to very young children, pregnant women, and lactating mothers.

These oils are not recommended to people who have fragrance allergies or sensitivities.

Rosemary.

Pros: Rosemary essential oils have analgesic, anti-inflammatory, and antispasmodic properties. It helps boost the immune system, improves overall mood, stimulate better circulation, speed up epidermal healing and slow down premature skin aging.

Best for: relieving back pains, especially in the lower lumbar area. This essential oil is also great in relieving headaches, joint pains, and muscle strains. It is commonly used to relieve sore muscles in the calves, ankles, feet, and toes.

However, the best use for rosemary essential oils is to promote better looking skin.

Cons: not recommended to people who have basil or mint allergies and sensitivities.

<u>**Sage**</u>. Clary sage.

Pros: contains anti-bacterial, antifungal, anti-inflammatory, antioxidant, antiseptic, and antispasmodic properties. It also has mild laxative properties. Sage essential oils relieves and/or reduces toxins in the body due to overconsumption of alcohol, fatty food items, salty food, and edibles with high sugar content.

Best for: full body massages. Sage essential oils promote healthy and young looking skin. It contains high levels of antioxidants and *cicastrisant* which lessens or slows down the emergence of skin spots, minor blemishes, wrinkles, and epidermal scars.

With the right application (and medical supervision,) sage essential oils can quickly heal incisions and wounds.

Sage essential oils also help relieve stress and anxiety.

Cons: sage is a stimulant, which makes this unsuitable for people with epilepsy, and those with nervous disorders. This is not recommended to children, pregnant women, and lactating mothers.

This must only be administered in small doses.

Sandalwood.

Pros: has anti-inflammatory, anti-spasmodic and sedative properties.

Best for: application on minor or superficial wounds, like: blemishes, insect bites, and scratches. Sandalwood essential oils also have trace amounts of *carminative* which is a natural muscle relaxant. This, plus its sedative property can induce relaxation, and ease anxiety and stress.

Studies show that sandalwood essential oil can reduce nerve pain and muscle strain.

Cons: Use sparingly around children, pregnant women, and lactating mothers.

Spruce.

Pros: this contains powerful sedative properties that work well as muscle relaxants.

Best for: easing some of the painful symptoms of arthritis, swollen lymph glands/nodes, lumbago, rheumatism, and *sciatica*.

Cons: spruce essential oils are relatively expensive due to its rarity in the open market. Also, because of its sedative properties, it can cause drowsiness, and is not recommended for day time use.

This is not recommended to young children, pregnant women, and lactating mothers.

Thyme. Red thyme. White thyme.

Pros: has anti-fungal, antiseptic and antispasmodic properties. It also contains trace amounts of stimulants that boost the immune system, stimulate better blood flow that improves cardiovascular functions, and ultimately relieve stress.

Best for: promoting better blood circulation, and for manual lymphatic drainage. Upper body massage using thyme essential oils helps improve respiratory and cardiovascular functions.

It can relieve some of the symptoms of asthma, bronchitis, blocked sinuses, colds, congestion, influenza, and seasonal allergies.

Cons: thyme essential oils must be used sparingly or in moderation. Too much can cause skin irritation.

This is not recommended to children, pregnant women, and lactating mothers.

This is also not for people with pre-existing skin conditions, or those who have highly sensitive skin.

Those who have basil or mint allergies or sensitivities can use these in small doses.

Vetiver.

Pros: has anti-inflammatory and antiseptic properties.

Best for: treating headaches and muscular pain. It also treats some of the symptoms of arthritis, gout, and rheumatism. Vetiver essential oils have been used for centuries in the east to strengthen connective tissues, improve circulatory functions, and prevent early bone loss.

This is great for treating cracked or dry skin.

Cons: These oils are not recommended to people who have fragrance allergies or sensitivities.

Do not use on children.

Wintergreen.

Pros: has analgesic, anti-rheumatic, anti-arthritic, antiseptic, and antispasmodic properties.

Best for: treating headaches and nerve pain. It can also ease symptoms of menstrual cramps, rheumatism, and arthritis. It can help lessen gout and lymph nodes swelling.

Small amounts of wintergreen essential oils can quickly heal superficial epidermal wounds like insect bites, scrapes, scratches, and open sores.

Cons: wintergreen essential oils should **never** be used for aromatherapy.

It should be used as topical solution diluted well in other oils or liquids. Use sparingly especially in the presence of children, pregnant women, and lactating mothers.

People with epileptic history should also avoid using wintergreen essential oils.

These oils are not recommended to people who have fragrance allergies or sensitivities.

Yarrow.

Pros: Yarrow essential oils have properties similar to chamomile extracts, and more. Aside from having anti-inflammatory properties, it also has anti-rheumatic, astringent, antiseptic and anti-spasmodic properties.

Best for: easing cramps, and muscles spasms. These oils also ease headaches and migraines as well as abdominal cramps brought about by PMS.

These work great for joint aches and muscle pains.

These help prevent constipation.

Cons: These must be used sparingly, and are not recommended for very young children, pregnant women, and lactating mothers. Use sparingly.

Some people are allergic to yarrow flowers/leaves. So if you experience headaches or any form of skin irritation after using yarrow essential oils, it would be best to wash it off immediately with soap and water. Yarrow allergy is not fatal.

3 Ways of Administering Essential Oils

If you are using essential oils to treat chronic pain, there are only 3 ways on how you can administer these on yourself or your loved ones. (Not including ingestion or consumption which is a different topic altogether.)

- Topical solutions. These are applied directly to the skin, and usually come in different forms, like: creams, foams, gels, lotions, ointments, and liquid soaps. If you prefer making your own topical solutions using your own essential oil blends, always remember to:

    o Dilute, dilute, and dilute your essential oil blends, especially fragrant ones. Really, it takes only one precious drop to make a cupful of lotion or creams.

    o Choose hypoallergenic and unscented mixing creams, foams, gels, lotions, ointments, and liquid soaps. This is to prevent scents from clashing.

    o Always do a skin test or patch test first before proceeding with the massage. This is essential if you already have prior allergies to other kinds of topical solutions.

    o Always use clean containers when mixing your blends.

o Always take careful not on what essential oils you are adding to your topical solutions, and the exact amount per mix.

- Aerial diffusion. This is to enhance or disinfect the environment you are working in. Essential oils or aromatic compounds are steamed or sprayed into the air, usually using a diffuser.

- Direct inhalation is used for respiratory disinfection, decongestion of the sinuses, or to promote expectoration. This should always be done under the supervision of a health care provider.

Tips on How to Buy Essential Oils

1. Always buy essential oils stored in glass bottles or glass dispensers. Never buy oils in plastic containers. Many essential oils become contaminated when stored in plastic bottles or jars, especially when these are exposed to sunlight, or to any heat source that has higher-than-body-temperature.

2. The best essential oils are stored in dark, amber glass containers. This prevents direct sunlight from affecting the quality of the oil. Avoid clear coloured bottles. Always opt for the dark, tinted, or coloured containers instead.

3. Always check product labels (or online product descriptions) before buying. High quality essential oils always have the least amount of ingredients listed. If possible, choose the ones with more natural ingredients, than artificially made ones.

4. Single or compound oils? Here is the low-down:

   Single oils or pure oils are usually those come from one source only. For example: pure wintergreen oil comes purely from steaming then processing the leaves of the wintergreen shrub. This usually comes out in concentrated formulas. This must be diluted first, or mixed with other liquids or oils.

Pure oils cannot be used as they are. These have to be mixed with other ingredients to make them less toxic to the skin or the lungs.

On the other hand, compound or complex wintergreen oil is pure wintergreen oil that is already diluted with other ingredients, like water or other kinds of oil, or mixed with other herbs, etc. This kind of product is almost always ready to use.

5. Always consider your allergies. Some people are sensitive to any kind of non-organic fragrance. They break out in spots when they come in contact with artificially-made fragrances or scent compounds. Others experience difficulty in breathing, and may even trigger asthma-like attacks. If you have this condition, always choose unscented massage oils.

   Also, some people are allergic to flower extracts and nuts. If you have a similar condition, avoid massage oils that contain tree nut (almond) or ground nut (peanut) oils. Also avoid ragweed (chamomile) extracts.

   To be safe, look for massage oils that specifically say: hypoallergenic.

6. Choose heavy oils for low friction massages (e.g. Swedish massage,) and light oils for high friction (e.g. deep tissue massages.)

Heavy massage oils (e.g. undiluted avocado oil, coconut oil, olive oil, peanut oil, sesame oil, etc.) take a long time to permeate through the skin. These are perfect for long and relaxing massages. These are also good for home or self-massages because of the small amount of heat they give off when rubbed on the skin or scalp.

These are not good for outdoor massages because these take a long time to wash out with soap and water. Plus, if it's warm outside, the oils will heat up as well.

Light massage oils (e.g. almond oil, cocoa butter, grapeseed oil, jojoba oil, shea butter, wheat germ oil, etc.) give just the right amount of lubrication for intense but short deep tissue massages without irritating the epidermis, or heating up the body.

Light massage oils are also quickly absorbed by the skin, which makes these easier to use outdoors, or for quick massage sessions.

7. Choose essential oils that have specific ingredients for specific body aches. When used correctly, any kind of massage oil will work on almost all kinds of chronic pain. But certain ingredients help speed up the healing process by several degrees.

* All images are from
www.pixabay.com

Conclusion

Thank you again and congratulations for finishing the book *"Anti-Inflammatory Essential Oils (18 Best Essential Oils For Inflammation)*

I hope you get a better insight as to why chronic pain happens, and how you can use organic, natural, and safe measures (such as using essential oils for simple massages) to help relieve some, if not all of its symptoms. The next step is to actually apply some of these measures to suit your own personal needs.

Any person living with chronic pain knows that any relief, big or small, is always worth pursuing. In this case, healing through the use of essential oils is a far better option than being a life-long dependent on drugs and other medications. Additionally, using massages to relieve one's pain is also 100% safer than undergoing any form of surgery or operation.

If you came this far, there's one way you can a make a difference: please review it on Amazon,com

Thank you once more. Have a wonderful pain-free day today!

www.ingramcontent.com/pod-product-compliance
Lightning Source LLC
Chambersburg PA
CBHW070301290526
45791CB00003B/1039